Understanding
Child Obesity &
The Essential Role
of Parents

Understanding Child Obesity & The Essential Role of Parents

Selva Sugunendran

CEng, MIEE, MCMI, CHt, MIMDHA, MBBNLP, MABNLP

#1 Best Selling Author, Speaker & "Success Through Wellness" Coach

To order additional copies of this book, contact:
Xlibris Corporation
0-800-644-6988
www.xlibrispublishing.co.uk
Orders@xlibrispublishing.co.uk
303645

CONTENTS

DEDICATION

This book is dedicated to all children (whether they are currently obese or not) and their parents, so that they can work as a team to fight against child obesity.

It is hoped that they will do so by choosing the Disease Prevention path called Wellness Solutions in preference to sickness-based treatment of symptoms, ensuring long term health and wellbeing.

This book is also dedicated to all others who have chosen this new golden path to better health and wellbeing.

"I continue to believe that if children are given the necessary tools to succeed, they will succeed beyond their wildest dreams!"

—David Vitter, U.S. Senator

DISCLAIMER AND COPYRIGHT

Every effort has been made to ensure the accuracy and completeness of the content provided in this book. However, the author, or any person associated with this book makes no warranties or guarantees, expressed or implied, regarding errors or omissions and assumes no legal liability or responsibility for loss or damage resulting from the use of information contained within.

Additionally, the author, or any person associated with this book does not guarantee, expressed or implied, for the accuracy, completeness, or usefulness of any information, apparatus, product, or process disclosed, or represents that its use would guarantee improvement or success in relation to subject written.

Any reference herein to any specific commercial products, processes, or services by trade name, trademark, manufacturer, or otherwise, does not necessarily constitute or imply its endorsement, recommendation, or favoring. The views of the author, or any other person associated with this book expressed herein are his or her own, based on personal experience.

The content of "Understanding Child Obesity & The Essential Role of Parents" is copyright protected, with all rights reserved and may not be copied or imitated in whole or part without first requesting and receiving full written permission from the author/owner.

Medical Disclaimer: The author of this e-book is a competent, experienced writer. He has taken every opportunity to ensure all information presented here is correct and up to date at the time of writing. No documentation within this book has been evaluated by the Food and Drug Administration, and no documentation should be used to diagnose, treat, cure, or prevent any disease.

Any information is to be used for educational and information purposes only. It should never be substituted for the medical advice from your own doctor or other health care professionals.

We do not dispense medical advice, prescribe drugs or diagnose any illnesses with our literature.

The author and publisher are not responsible or liable for any self or third party diagnosis made by visitors based upon the content in this book. Neither does the author or publisher in any way endorse any commercial products or services linked from other websites to this book.

Please, always consult your doctor or health care specialist if you are in any way concerned about your physical wellbeing.

INTRODUCTION

For children living with obesity, not only is there the challenge associated with what society deems to be unacceptable appearance but even more importantly, increasing health risks. Child obesity is a growing epidemic in many parts of the world and for the children caught up in it life can be very difficult. In this book, we want to address the dynamics of child obesity, provide reasons why this problem develops, and show the key role that parents play in preventing and eliminating the problem.

It is important to understand that even though child obesity is becoming more and more prevalent and serious, a variety of tools, resources, and healthcare treatments are currently available to help. For the children who are picked on, teased, and have to deal with ongoing health problems associated with obesity, they need to know that this problem is not a life sentence of misery.

Change is possible and while it requires hard work, determination, and a solid support system provided by the parents, as well as siblings, friends, and teachers, obese children can enjoy life to its fullest. The key to understanding child obesity is education! For this reason, we have provided information not only the different reasons why children become obese but also a working plan to help children lose weight and adopt a healthier lifestyle. With proper diet and exercise, the body can be transformed.

It is common for obese children to drop the weight but unfortunately, some are left with psychological scars because of the many years of torment. Parents are vital players in the process of educating children and helping them recapture their youth through a healthy body and mind. Because of this, the book is written for obese children and the parents so they can work as a team along with receiving support from a qualified doctor to fight against child obesity!

IMPORTANT MESSAGE TO PARENTS

For most parents, two rules of parenting apply:

1. There is no official parenting handbook
2. Parents are like bears, fighting to protect children at any cost

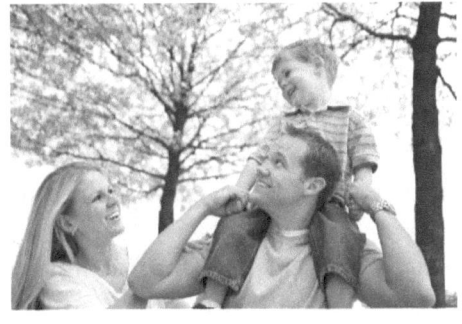

We wanted to begin this book with a message to parents since several things within this book are tough to hear. It is vital that parents of obese children stop carrying around a black cloud of guilt. Child obesity is a condition that affects literally millions of children all over the world, a condition caused by a variety of things.

Using the two rules listed above, we felt it was important to stress a couple of issues specific to each.

Parenting Handbook

Yes, you can read numerous books such as this, watch DVDs, listen to CDs, read magazines, participate in parenting classes, and even attend seminars but because every child on the face of the planet is unique, no single handbook is going to work. Remember, each child has his or her own personality, characteristics traits, family history, physical makeup, and opinions. Trying to capture all the dynamics in one resource would be *impossible*.

The reason this is important is that regardless of how well a parent raises a child, mistakes are going to happen. Every parent has to make choices believed to be in the best interest of the child but again, with so many different factors involved, each child will respond differently. If you have an obese child, perhaps you could have made better choices regarding diet and physical activity but good parenting means to learn, make corrections or adjustments, and keep striving for the best!

Parents are Bears

This does not mean parents are grumpy, but experts agree that of all wild animals on the planet, bears are the most protective of their young. Good parents are much the same, doing anything in their power to keep their child safe, happy, and healthy. Therefore, if you are a parent of an obese child, in no way did you intentionally do something purposely to create the challenges surrounding this condition.

All parents reflect at some point, only to realize that perhaps they could have made wiser choices. As a parent of an obese child your number one goal is to provide every opportunity for your child. To combat the problem of obesity, you and the child can work as a team to learn from the past, address the areas that need to be improved on, and then take a proactive approach to change.

We want to emphasize to every parent reading this book that the intention of writing it is not to criticize or judge—period! Instead, the focus of this book is to help educate parents and children about the potential risks that go along with child obesity, why children can end up in this situation, and different steps that can be taken to leave the past alone and start to focus on a bright and healthy future.

In saying that, as you read some of the tougher areas, do not take them as a personal attack. In fact, you have no reason to feel defensive in that all parents have areas of raising a child that could be done better. Therefore, please understand we support parents of obese children and understand this subject is very sensitive. We welcome you to take the information that pertains to your specific situation and apply it so you can prevent or get the condition of obesity under control.

Parenting is tough—whether dealing with a physically disabled child, one with a learning disability, a teenager going through a rebellious stage, or managing a situation of a child with obesity. We applaud you for reaching out to become educated and for allowing us to introduce you to information, tools, and resources that can be used in the battle against this worldwide epidemic.

This book was not written to challenge the intelligence or integrity of parents but to remind all of us that great parenting means loving a child unconditionally and unselfishly. Helping an obese child transition from a current lifestyle to one that will bring the challenge of obesity under control will take a tremendous amount of love and patience but we are 100% confident you will succeed!

"I continue to believe that if children are given the necessary tools to succeed, they will succeed beyond their wildest dreams!"

David Vitter, U.S. Senator

OVERVIEW OF CHILD OBESITY

Before we do anything else, it is important to understand the basics of child obesity. After all, many parents realize their child is overweight but have never considered that the child falls within the range of obesity. Although it is unhealthy anytime a child carries around any extra weight, once weight and body mass (fat) reaches a certain point, the situation becomes critical.

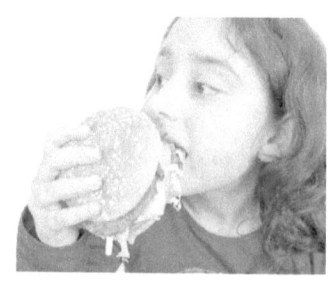

As you will discover, a thin line exists between a child just being heavy and a child being obese. The greatest concern is that once a child has reached the level of obesity the potential for health risks increases significantly. The frightening thing about child obesity is that it can happen so quickly. Obviously, prevention is always the best course but for children already dealing with this condition it is essential for parents and children to become educated.

Although many cases of obesity can be avoided, not all can. For instance, this condition can be found in children who have been raised on the wrong type and quantities of food from a very young age. For this reason, educating parents about proper diet and nutrition is a great preventative tool. Once a child's weight reaches a point where the Body Mass Index or BMI exceeds 30, the child is officially diagnosed as being obese.

While obesity is not a new problem, it has become far more prevalent in just the past 10 years all over the world. Although all countries deal with child obesity on some level, statistics show that some countries have a much larger problem than other countries. For instance, children being raised in the United States and the United Kingdom are among those at greatest risk.

Although a lot of information has been disseminated to the public in recent years about prevention, causes, and risks associated with child obesity, many people still view this condition as being more cosmetic than health-related. The truth is that child obesity goes deeper that outward appearance. This condition actually increases a variety of health risks and it can have a negative impact on the child's psychological health.

Studies show that many children with obesity deal with emotional and mental issues long after losing weight. From a physical standpoint, if left untreated, obesity can cause a number of healthy problems, even major organ damage. This is why becoming educated and getting the child the best treatment possible specific to physical and psychological health is so crucial.

Consider that a significant amount of weight puts tremendous strain on the body's organs, bones, and joints for anyone but this is extremely difficult for children who are still in the growing stage. As an example, added weight to the bones of an adult is a challenge but when excess weight is put on bones of children whose bones are still growing and developing and thereby not that strong, different problems can occur.

The information provided in this book is designed to help enlighten parents and children to the true effects associated with child obesity. It is important to understand that knowledge is power and with power, change is possible. The need to educate entire families and communities about child obesity has become urgent. The sooner potential risks are fully understood—the sooner appropriate changes can be made.

Education is a powerful tool, one that provides parents with an excellent opportunity to leave the past behind and start moving forward with a healthier lifestyle consisting of nutritional meals and fun physical activity.

WORLDWIDE STATISTICS

Most parents are shocked when they learn the statistics associated with child obesity. While most people are aware of this problem the truth is that many have never grasped the full scope. To show parents just how serious child obesity is, we have provided research to show how this condition affects the lives of millions of children all over the world.

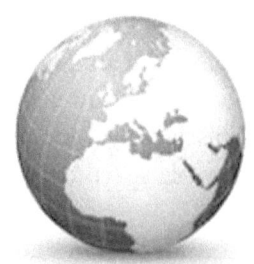

We felt it was important to point to some of the countries where child obesity is virtually unknown, as well as countries where child obesity has reached epidemic proportions. As an example, throughout the United States and the United Kingdom, child obesity numbers are extremely high. Because this condition affects so many families, global health officials have begun to take a more aggressive approach to prevention and cure.

Over the past several years, a number of new strategies have been developed to combat child obesity but most have been on the level of the child and parents. While it certainly helps families to be educated about poor diet and improper physical activity, the truth is that entire communities need the same education. One organization[1] is spearheading something far more comprehensive, as it reaches out to food producers, enlisting them to stake a claim in producing and packaging healthier food items.

We are all concerned with the increasing cost of healthcare and the impact this has had on insurance coverage but unfortunately, child obesity is a

---

[1]   World Health Organization

contributor to the problem. The reason—obesity is directly linked to several major health conditions to include heart disease, hypertension, diabetes, and others.

As a result, anytime a child's health is compromised due to obesity, it means more trips to the doctor and more in-depth treatments are required. Because of this, the parent's health insurance company pays out larger sums of money for these additional health problems that would otherwise not need financial coverage.

Although there are many astounding facts relating to child obesity, one that leaves us perplexed is that even in third-world countries were malnutrition and even starvation are serious problems, obese children can be found. This just shows that the problem of child obesity has no boundaries.

Impact on Foreign Countries

Another organization[2] has spent countless hours of hard work to identify, gather, and compile facts about child obesity in foreign countries. This research shows that approximately 22 million children worldwide under the age of five are either overweight or actually obese.

As an example, research has been conducted in various regions of Africa and the results show that the problem of overweight and obese children is more prevalent than malnutrition is. In fact, research shows that the ratio of overweight/obesity to malnutrition on this continent is now 4 to 1. In other words, 0.7% of children in Africa were undernourished whereas 3% were overweight or obese!

Some additional details that have come out of various studies done on child obesity around the world include:

- Globally, approximately 750 million people are overweight and another 300 million obese. Of these, a large percentage is children.

---

[2]   International Obesity Task Force

- Egypt—Up to 25% of children four years and younger are overweight or obese
- Mexico, Chile, and Peru—Up to 25% of children between the ages of four and ten are overweight or obese
- Morocco and Zambia—Between 15% and 20% of children four years and younger are obese
- In foreign countries, the primary contributor to child obesity is junk food

Impact on the United States

Within the United States, a diagnosis of child obesity is typically provided when the child's total body weight is comprised of 25% fat for boys and 32% fat for girls. This means when a child has a BMI in the 95th percentile specific to age and gender using the growth chart provided by the Centers for Disease Control and Prevention, a diagnosis of obesity would be made.

Since 2000, several in-depth studies have been conducted specific to child obesity. These studies have provided a real look into this problem and while numbers are currently at epidemic proportions, are some countries are starting to see a decline in diagnoses. Some of the findings gathered over the past few years include the following:

- In the United States, close to 15% of obese people are children and in other countries, the numbers climb to 30%
- One of every seven preschool children living in a low-income family is obese. The number of confirmed cases between two and four years of age specific to low-income families has increased by almost 15% from 1998 to 2008.
- Children of Alaskan Native or American Indian descent are among the fastest growing groups for child obesity, which rose about one-half percent from 2003 to 2008
- The breakdown of child obesity for different ethnic groups in the United States includes:

  ○ Alaskan Native and American Indian—21.2%
  ○ Hispanic—18.5%
  ○ Pacific Islander and Asian—12.3%

- African American—11.8%
- Children living in Colorado and Hawaii—Less than 10%

Potential Risk

Potential risk of children moving from being overweight to being obese has increased. Knowing these facts can help parents recognize potential for a child battling weight to become obese. At that point, parents can take preventative measures.

- From 1980 to 2010, the percentage of overweight children between the ages of six and eleven rose by 50%
- From 1994 to 2001, the percentage of children between the ages of two and five rose by 42%

Additional Health Factors

Because we know that obese children are at an increased risk of developing serious health problems, ongoing studies are being conducted to determine the real impact of this condition. The following information came out of one of the latest studies, which is alarming.

- Of children diagnosed with Type 2 diabetes, 20% can be linked directly to obesity
- Of children with early warning signs associated with Type 2 diabetes, approximately 25% are overweight
- Of overweight children, about 60% have at least one risk factor for heart disease
- Of children with a firm diagnosis of Type 2 diabetes, 85% are overweight

Statistics on Additional Countries

The following table shows statistics for adult obesity but in foreign countries, 25% to 30% are children and in North America, approximately 15% are children.

NORTH AMERICA	
Country	**Total Obesity Statistics** *M=Million* *T=Thousands*
United States	43 M
Canada	4.8 M
Mexico	15.4 M

CENTRAL AMERICA	
Country	**Total Obesity Statistics** *M=Million* *T=Thousands*
Belize	40 T
Guatemala	2.1 M
Nicaragua	785 T

CARIBBEAN	
Country	**Total Obesity Statistics** *M=Million* *T=Thousands*
Puerto Rico	570 T

SOUTH AMERICA	
Country	**Total Obesity Statistics** *M=Million* *T=Thousands*
Brazil	27 M
Chile	2.3 M
Colombia	6.2 M

Paraguay	906 T
Peru	4 M
Venezuela	3.7 M

NORTHERN EUROPE	
Country	**Total Obesity Statistics** *M=Million* *T=Thousands*
Denmark	792 T
Finland	753 T
Iceland	43 T
Sweden	1.3 M

WESTERN EUROPE	
Country	**Total Obesity Statistics** *M=Million* *T=Thousands*
Belgium	1.5 M
France	8.8 M
Ireland	581 T
Monaco	4.8 T
Netherlands	2.4 M
United Kingdom	8.8 M
Wales	427 T

CENTRAL EUROPE	
Country	Total Obesity Statistics M=Million T=Thousands
Austria	1.2 M
Czech Republic	182 T
Germany	12.1 M
Hungary	1.5 M
Poland	5.7 M
Slovakia	794 T
Slovenia	294 T
Switzerland	1.1 M

EASTERN EUROPE	
Country	Total Obesity Statistics M=Million T=Thousands
Belarus	1.5 M
Estonia	196 T
Latvia	337 T
Lithuania	528 T
Russia	21.1 M
Ukraine	7 M

SOUTHWEST EUROPE	
Country	**Total Obesity Statistics** *M=Million* *T=Thousands*
Azerbaijan	1.2 M
Georgia	687 T
Portugal	1.6 M
Spain	5.9 M

SOUTHERN EUROPE	
Country	**Total Obesity Statistics** *M=Million* *T=Thousands*
Greece	1.6 M
Italy	8.4 M

SOUTHEAST EUROPE	
Country	**Total Obesity Statistics** *M=Million* *T=Thousands*
Albania	519 T
Bosnia/Herzegovina	60 T
Bulgaria	1.1 M
Croatia	658 T
Macedonia	299 T
Romania	3.2 M
Serbvia/Montenegro	1.6 M

NORTHERN ASIA	
Country	**Total Obesity Statistics** **M=Million** **T=Thousands**
Mongolia	403 T

CENTRAL ASIA	
Country	**Total Obesity Statistics** **M=Million** **T=Thousands**
Kazakhstan	2.2 M
Tajikistan	1.1 M
Uzbekistan	3.9 M

EASTERN ASIA	
Country	**Total Obesity Statistics** **M=Million** **T=Thousands**
China	190 M
Hong Kong	1 M
Japan	19 M
Macau	65 T
N. Korea	3.3 M
S. Korea	7.1 M
Taiwan	3.3 M

SOUTHWEST ASIA	
Country	**Total Obesity Statistics** *M=Million* *T=Thousands*
Turkey	10.1 M

SOUTHERN ASIA	
Country	**Total Obesity Statistics** *M=Million* *T=Thousands*
Afghanistan	4.2 M
Bangladesh	21 M
Bhutan	320 T
India	156 M
Pakistan	24 M
Sri Lanka	3 M

SOUTHEAST ASIA	
Country	**Total Obesity Statistics** *M=Million* *T=Thousands*
Indonesia	35 T
Laos	888 T
Malaysia	3.5 M
Philippines	13 M
Singapore	637 T
Thailand	9.4 M
Vietnam	12.1 M

CENTRAL AMERICA	
Country	**Total Obesity Statistics** *M=Million* *T=Thousands*
Belize	40 T
Guatemala	2 M
Nicaragua	79 T

MIDDLE EAST	
Country	**Total Obesity Statistics** *M=Million* *T=Thousands*
Gaza Strip	194 T
Iran	9.9 M
Iraq	3.7 M
Israel	907 T
Jordan	821 T
Kuwait	330 T
Lebanon	553 T
Saudi Arabia	3.7 M
Syria	2.6 M
United Arab Emirates	369 T
West Bank	338 T
Yemen	2.9 M

NORTH AFRICA	
Country	**Total Obesity Statistics** *M=Million* *T=Thousands*
Egypt	11 M
Libya	824 T
Sudan	5.7 M

WEST AFRICA	
Country	**Total Obesity Statistics** *M=Million* *T=Thousands*
Congo Brazzaville	439 T
Ghana	3 M
Liberia	496 T
Niger	1.7 M
Nigeria	2.6 M
Senegal	1.6 M
Sierra Leone	861 T

CENTRAL AFRICA	
Country	**Total Obesity Statistics** *M=Million* *T=Thousands*
Central African Republic	548 T
Chad	1.4 M
Congo Kinshasa	8.5 M
Rwanda	1.2 M

EAST AFRICA	
Country	**Total Obesity Statistics** *M=Million* *T=Thousands*
Ethiopia	10 M
Kenya	4.8 M
Somalia	1.2 M
Tanzania	5.2 M
Uganda	3.9 M

SOUTH AFRICA	
Country	**Total Obesity Statistics** *M=Million* *T=Thousands*
Angola	1.6 M
Botswana	240 T
South Africa	6.5 M
Swaziland	171 T
Zambia	1.6 M
Zimbabwe	537 T

OCEANIA	
Country	**Total Obesity Statistics** *M=Million* *T=Thousands*
Australia	2.9 M
New Zealand	584 T
Papua New Guinea	793 T

CAUSES OF CHILD OBESITY

As we mentioned, one of the main causes of child obesity is directly linked to poor diet. However, as you will discover in this chapter, a child can develop this problem from other causes.

As a part of the educational journey, it is critical to learn all the different causes so proper changes can be made immediately, perhaps preventing a case of child obesity or bringing the condition under control.

Keep in mind that the causes listed are only those that have to date been identified. Because of child obesity being such a serious and growing issue, a significant amount of research money and time has been put into identifying all the causes, as well as developing new medication and/or treatment.

Improper Diet

Because improper diet is a huge contributor to child obesity, we want to touch on it first. The formula for dealing with child obesity is that the number of calories consumed daily must decrease and the level of physical activity done daily must increase. By providing the child with different food choices, you can actually increase the amount of food while at the same time reducing his or her caloric intake.

The formula for calorie consumption versus calories burned is actually simple. A single pound is equivalent to 3,500 calories. Throughout the day, the body naturally burns calories for breathing, walking, and even sitting. The stored calories are burned as fuel, or energy.

A prime example of how weight is lost, consider the following:

- Consumption of 1,500 calories a day (7 x 1,500 = 10,500 calories weekly)
- Regular calorie burning by the body plus physical activity burns 2,500 a day (7 x 2,500 = 17,500 calories weekly)
- Total calories consumed weekly minus total calories burned weekly (10,500—17,500 =—7,000)
- The—7,000 is divided by 3,500 (one calorie) for a total of—2, which means within a one-week period using this formula, a child would drop approximately 2 pounds

This formula shows that to lose weight, the doctor would need to determine the appropriate number of calories consumed on a daily basis, which would be different for each child since it is based on individual factors. Additionally, the doctor could provide some great options for age-appropriate physical activity or you could research options on your own.

Studies show that most obese children consume on average 1,000 calories a day beyond what the body requires. Then for calories burned, this is based on a number of factors but for a sedentary lifestyle, the average is 1,700. Regarding the actual number of calories a child needs, consider this statistic.

Typically by age one a child requires 1,000 calories and for each year of life thereafter, 200 calories would be added until age 13 so by the time a girl and boy is in their mid-teens, the total number of calories needed daily are between 2,200 and 3,000 respectively.

Using the same formula provided above, if a six-year old child that required 1,200 calories a day but who was consuming 2,200 and only burning the average 1,700 calories, means that child would be gaining a full pound every week! The problem with many diets today is that they include fatty and high-caloric snacks that children do not need. Even worse than the actual food, snacks and even meals are being consumed while watching television, playing video games, or spending time on the computer.

If a child lives this type of lifestyle, it would only be a matter of time before he or she would begin to gain weight. Once a child starts putting on weight, the pounds quickly begin to pile on and before a parent even realizes, the child has passed that thin line that separates being heavy into the world of child obesity.

Lack of Physical Activity

Even if a child were eating a healthy diet, if he or she were not getting any physical activity, high risk for obesity would exist. Some children avoid participating in sports or other physical activity due to shyness or there may be physical limitations associated with another health problem.

The good news is that with physical activity being such a critical part of a child's health, we now see incredible programs being developed or already offered for children of all ages. Parents need to scout out activities that would interest the child and then provide full support in getting him or her started.

In fact, one of the best ways of encouraging an obese child to participate in physical activity is for the entire family to join in. No matter the choice, being involved with activities together provides support needed by the child while benefiting the entire family.

Just a few examples of physical activity that children and the rest of the family could do together include:

- Martial Arts
- Dance
- Swimming
- Biking
- Hiking
- Bowling

Genetics

While not as common, some genetic problems can cause child obesity. If a child were eating a nutritional diet and getting physical activity but the parent notices he or she is putting on weight quickly, a doctor who specializes in child obesity should determine why. In many cases, something can be done to stop the weight gain before it gets out of hand.

Although more research is needed, some new evidence is being identified whereby flawed DNA may be linked to child obesity. Researchers from two British organizations[3] took DNA from overweight or obese children around the age of 10 who weighed around 220 pounds and examined it. For this, the primary focus was on additional or missing DNA segments.

These researchers discovered that a number of rare missing segments might in fact be responsible for promoting child obesity. One deletion in particular was found in less than 1% of about 1,200 children participating in the study. Interestingly, the deletion had nothing to do with slowing down metabolism but actually causing an increase in hunger.

The missing segment of the DNA was found on chromosome 16 and what made this discovery so significant was that this flawed segment actually eliminated a specific gene required by the brain for producing Leptin, an appetite-suppressing hormone. As one doctor put it, without this gene, a person would constantly be hungry even if he or she recently ate. As a result, fast weight gain would be expected.

Age

Although rare, when a child begins to enter the years of puberty, a time when hormones are raging, obesity can develop. Typically, obesity associated with age would be seen in adults but it is a possibility for teenagers as well.

Financial Lifestyle

Interestingly, studies also show that affluent families, those that travel often, lavish the children with gifts, and have all the luxuries that money can afford often have at least one obese child. In this case, experts believe a number of factors could be the reason. For instance, affluent families are

---

[3]   University of Cambridge/Wellcome Trust Sanger Institute

often on the go, which means they grab food from fancy restaurants that serve rich, high caloric foods.

In addition, many families with money often have an intent focus on the things they can buy for their children such as toys, clothing, gadgets, trips, etc, but for some children on the receiving end, they feel immense pressure that in return, they must perfect. Because of this, some children turn to the comfort of food as a method of dealing with what they perceive to be the expectation of excelling or surpassing expectations of the parents.

Family History

Since obesity can run in families, not just because of a genetic link, but unhealthy habits specific to poor diet, lack of physical activity, and even lifestyle, children may follow the parent's example. If one parent has been or is currently obese, the child has an increased risk for being obese but if both parents were or are obese, risk of the child developing obesity increases dramatically.

Medication

While uncommon, certain medications can actually cause child obesity or enhance other things that cause this condition. Of course, any concerns specific to medication would need to be addressed with the child's doctor but the most common drugs that promote child obesity include those used to treat various psychiatric conditions and steroid hormones.

Regardless of the reason a child has developed obesity, it is vital that this condition is never ignored. It is important for the child to get a firm diagnosis and for parents to develop a strategy that will not only help the child lose weight and regain confidence but something that would benefit the entire family.

Instead of looking at child obesity as a hopeless situation, you could view it as an opportunity for the family to start eating better and participating in an activity that everyone enjoys!

DIAGNOSING CHILD OBESITY

Any parent with concerns regarding a child's health should have him or her checked by a doctor. If you as the parent suspected child obesity, it would be beneficial for the child to be seen by a doctor that specializes in this problem.

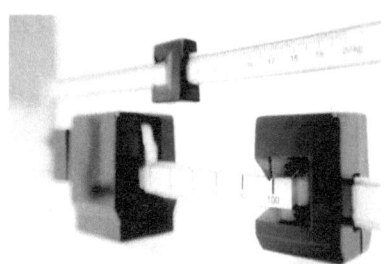

A doctor that commonly treats obese children is going to be more empathetic to the situation and have the most recent information regarding studies, medication, therapies, etc.

Choosing a Doctor

The first step would be to choose the right doctor. Some family doctors are highly qualified for treating child obesity but if not, he or she would be able to recommend a specialist or you could use any number of doctor referral services—a few are listed below. Additionally, parents could talk to the insurance company, asking if they could offer names of doctors covered by the policy.

- Metro Health—*http://www.metrohealth.org/body.cfm?id=2660*
- Memorial Healthcare System—*http://www.mhs.net/physicians*
- UCLA Physician Referral Service—*http://www.uclahealth.org/body.cfm?id=308*
- Cedars Sinai—*https://referrals.cedars-sinai.edu*

Once the doctor has been located, the child would then be taken in for a physical examination. If possible, it would be advantageous for both parents to go, which would show the child that he/she is being provided with full support. Whether the mom and dad, a single parent, or a guardian goes, sitting down with the doctor provides an opportunity to gain insight and ask questions.

Testing

Initially, the doctor would obtain a medical history of the child, followed by conducting a variety of tests so that a firm diagnosis could be made.

Weight

The child would step on a scale without shoes or heavy clothing items to be weighed. This number of pounds would then be listed in the child's medical file, later used to determine BMI.

Height

After being weighed, the child's height would be measured and recorded. The weight and height combined are what allow the doctor to determine an accurate BMI.

BMI

After going through questions pertaining to health history, the doctor would determine the child's BMI. While the number of pounds on the scale is important, the BMI is the most critical factor since it deals with percentage of body fat. The child's BMI would be identified using a specific formula as shown below:

- A BMI less than 18.5 shows the child to be underweight
- A BMI of 18.5 to 24.9 places the child in a normal or healthy range
- A BMI of 25.0 to 29.9 indicates the child is overweight
- A BMI of 30 or more confirms obesity

An example of how the equation of weight and height would be used to determine BMI includes the following:

- Child's weight (pounds) would be multiplied by 703 (i.e., a child weighing 230 pounds would produce a number of 161,690)
- Child's height in total number of inches would be multiplied by itself or squared (i.e., a child 64 inches tall would have a square number of 4,096)
- The child's multiplied weight number would be then divided by the squared height inches (i.e., 161,690 divided by 4,096 equals 39.48)
- The 39.48 is the child's BMI, offering a firm diagnosis of obesity

Growth Charts

In addition to BMI, most doctors now refer to a child growth chart that shows the appropriate height and weight for a child of a specific age. Additionally, these charts are broken down between male and female since there are some variances between genders. Based on the child's height and weight, the doctor would be able to see the percentile in which the child falls. This data would provide the doctor with valuable insight into the severity of the condition.

As an example, if a child was in the 70th percentile for weight, it would mean when compared to other children of the same age and gender, 70% of the other children have a lower BMI. To make it easier and more precise when diagnosing a child with obesity, specific cutoffs[4] have been established. These cutoffs are currently used by doctors along with the growth charts to include:

- If the BMI falls between the 85th and 95th percentiles, the child is considered overweight
- If the BMI falls above the 95th percentile, the child is considered obese

Knowing a child's BMI is crucial tool for making a firm diagnosis of obesity. However, along with using this number for making a diagnosis,

---

[4]   Centers for Disease Control and Prevention

it is important to understand that the BMI formula does not account for everything. For instance, a muscular child or one with a larger body structure than most children of the same age and gender would not have a fair weight assessment.

Because the doctor depends on BMI for diagnosis and treatment, when faced with unique scenarios, further evaluation would be required. When working with BMI numbers, the doctor would likely want to know about any family history of obesity, as well as any past or current health risks associated with excess weight to include heart disease, diabetes, high blood pressure, high cholesterol, etc.

The doctor would also want a full outline of the type and frequency of food the child eats and the total number of calories for the child on a daily basis. Additionally, the child's physical activity level would need to be added to the equation, along with any other health conditions.

All of these things combined are what allows a medical professional to diagnose a child with obesity. When that has been completed, a proactive strategy for getting the problem under control could be developed.

POSSIBLE RISKS AND COMPLICATIONS

In this chapter, we felt it was important to address some of the possible risks and complications that go along with child obesity. This information is not intended to scare parents or children but more to show the severity of this condition if not prevented or managed.

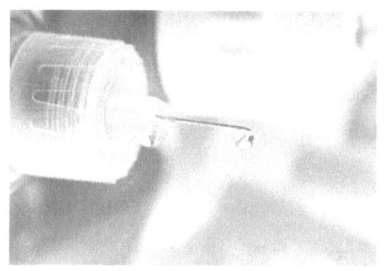

Sadly, children have died from complications associated with child obesity but in the majority of cases, proper intervention would have changed the outcome. Keep in mind that overweight children are also at risk but once the child reaches the level of obesity, the number of incidences for these risks and complications rise.

When anyone carries around a significant amount of weight, it is expected that the body is going to struggle since the body is not designed to handle this type of stress. For children, being overweight or obese only intensifies the potential for problems.

Health Problems

Below, we have listed some of the more specific issues that might be seen in children living with this condition.

- Blood Lipid Abnormalities (Fat)
- Cancer (rectal, colon, breast, uterine, cervix, ovarian, and prostate)

- Depression
- Gallbladder Disease
- Gynecological (infertility and/or irregular menstrual cycles)
- Heart Disease
- High Blood Pressure
- Metabolic Syndrome
- Nonalcoholic Fatty Liver Disease
- Osteoarthritis
- Skin Conditions (Intertrigo, which is an inflammatory condition found in skin folds due to excess moisture and/or slow wound healing)
- Sleep Apnea
- Stroke
- Type 2 Diabetes

Reduced Quality of Life

Child obesity can reduce quality of life from a physical and psychological standpoint. While some children do relatively well, others struggle. For instance, physical limitations are likely since carrying around excess weight is difficult. In this case, the child would experience slower movements, delayed development, and painful joints and muscles, as well as have a greater potential for injury.

From a psychological point of view, obesity often leads to a child being picked on and teased, or unable to participate in social events. With this, many children will begin to withdraw, which is seen a decreasing desire to spend time with friends, go to birthday parties, participate in family outings, and so on. In older children, some will start isolating themselves in the bedroom.

In addition to being withdrawn, sometimes as quality of life deteriorates in older children, parents will see the child starting to act out in a variety of ways such as dressing bizarre, becoming promiscuous, being rebellious, hanging out with a bad crowd, or failing in school.

When you notice a change in your child it means that he or she is beginning to have reduced quality of life from being obese. These are all warning signs that medical and parental intervention is imperative. Remember, as obese children age, they become more aware of ways the weight is affecting life. This can manifest in several ways to include:

- Depression
- Disability
- Physical Discomfort or Pain
- Shame and Embarrassment
- Social Isolation

Psychosocial Issues

As a parent, you need to expect that your child will end up dealing with some degree of psychosocial issue. Unfortunately, school age children can be downright cruel. As adults, we can rationalize that bullies in school are the kids who are really struggling from self-esteem issues and to boost their power and presence, they pick on easy targets. However, the obese child being teased and bullied, the outlook is very different.

Studies show that the younger the child is when the teasing begins the more challenging the psychosocial issues can be. Once an obese child is old enough to be aware of why the teasing and bullying is occurring he or she can feel extreme stress and even shame. In return, the child's sense of self-worth is altered and if no intervention is offered, this can become a very serious problem.

When a child begins to struggle with self-esteem and self-confidence, that child starts to question everything in life. Before long, parents notice the child's grades dropping and the number of friends dwindling. As a parent, these should be warning signs that immediate help is needed.

Sadly, when looking at adults who turn to drugs or lives of crime, most were children that suffered extreme teasing. This does not mean that every obese child who experiences being picked on is going to grow up to be a drug addict or criminal but it does shed some light on the importance of understanding that obese children are at greater risk.

MEDICAL INTERVENTION
AND TREATMENT

Proper treatment for obesity is also important. The doctor would begin by recommending that the child eat a healthier diet and get adequate physical activity but sometimes, medication and therapy is needed, as well.

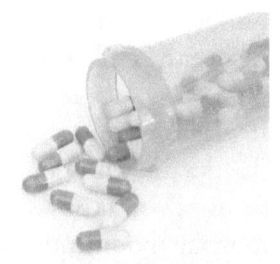

Toward the end of this book, we have offered some recommendations for dietary and physical activity books, as well as other resources that would be a huge benefit to both the parents and child. However, we also wanted to cover healthcare intervention in this chapter for the seriously obese child, especially one dealing with a secondary health risk.

Remember, with child obesity, not only do doctors need to treat the weight problem but also other health conditions relating to obesity such as those mentioned earlier. The best time for healthcare intervention is as soon as symptoms are noticed or a firm diagnosis of child obesity provided. Since obesity can lead to major problems, unless intervention and treatment are provided and parents become educated, the problem of obesity will only worsen.

At that time, obesity changes from a "problem" or "condition" to an actual disease. Today, doctors take child obesity very seriously and because of that children are receiving much better treatment than ever before. Doctors that specialize in child obesity know that it is just as important to educate the parents, providing them with management tools. Some of these are provided in the following chapter, tools that parents can use as a guide or reference.

From a medical standpoint, the exact medication and/or treatment provided to a child would depend on a number of factors. For instance, the child's age, level of obesity, degree of mobility, psychological stability, understanding, and additional health issues would all be considered.

Regardless of the type of medicine or treatment offered, the goal is always to reduce weight, which in turn would help lower the child's blood pressure, blood glucose levels, and cholesterol, as well as reduce risk of developing full-blown heart disease or Type 2 diabetes. Initially, a goal would be set to reduce the child's weight by 10%.

If weight were lost on the established treatment program, it would provide the doctor with confirmation that the appropriate course of action were being taken. If no weight were lost, the doctor would have the opportunity to make modifications.

Low Calorie Diet

The first change would consist of putting the child on a Low Calorie Diet, also referred to as LCD. This would reduce caloric intake by 500 to 1,000 depending on severity of the obesity. For younger children the change is relatively easy but for older kids there is more of a challenge. As a parent, you can learn ways to make this transition to healthier eating by substituting foods that still have flavor and make your child feel full quicker and longer.

For a child age seven and younger with obesity, but one without any secondary health risk, most doctors will simply create a weight management plan opposed to a weight loss plan. The reason is that by maintaining proper diet and physical activity, as the child grows the weight will be proportioned to height, thus falling within a normal range. On the other hand, weight loss programs are usually designed for children older than age seven.

Physical Activity Management

Next, the doctor would recommend an appropriate physical activity program for the child. The age of the child would determine how the ease in which this program would be introduced. Younger children are typically eager to get involved whereas older children may take a little more coaxing. As a parent, you can make it easier to incorporate physical activity into the child's life by using fun activity DVDs developed specifically for children with obesity.

In addition to weight loss, a good physical activity program would reduce body fat, which in turn improves cardiovascular fitness. Initially, the child should only stay active for about 20 minutes, three to four days a week. After a month, this could increase to 30 minutes, four days a week, and with two months, physical activity would be at 45 minutes to an hour five days a week.

To avoid aggravation, strain, or even injury to bones, joints, and tissues, it is important that the different types of physical activity be staggered. As an example, aerobic activity would be done three days a week such as swimming, biking, or playing tennis and two days a week, strength/muscle building activities. Of course, if a child complains of pain, parents should ease up or provide the child with a week off from physical activity to allow the body to rest.

Behavioral Therapy

After the low calorie diet plan and physical activity program have been established, the doctor would likely want the child to go through behavioral therapy. Parents need to understand this does not mean the child is mentally ill or even a bad person simply that he or she needs to be taught a new way of thinking, processing, and acting.

Obesity does not only affect the body but the mind too. Children who go through behavioral therapy understand that they are important and a viable part of society whether obese or not.

Medication

For treating child obesity, doctors can use both non-prescription and prescription medications. Typically, doctors start with something over-the-counter but if this does not help, prescribed medication is an alternative. Doctors seldom use non-prescription or prescription medication when treating small children.

While some medications can be beneficial for older children and teenagers, careful monitoring is vital. Usually, treatment for children 10 and younger involves education, diet, physical activity, and behavior modification without the use of any medication.

Non-Prescription

A number of non-prescription medications are now being used to treat obesity but not all can be offered to small children. However, for older children, Alli is one choice that has been considered effective and safe. This medication is formulated to stop fat associated with consumed food from being absorbed into the body.

Keep in mind that the version of non-prescription Alli has approval from the Food and Drug Administration but it is a reduced strength formula, not what you would find with prescription Alli. Even so, only children 18 and older are advised to take this over-the-counter version of Alli for treating obesity due to unpleasant side effects such as gas, bloating, and stomachache.

Prescription

The two primary types of prescription medication used for treating child obesity include orlistat, which is branded as Xenical or Alli and sibutramine, branded under the name of Meridia. A prescription of Meridia is only approved for children 16 and older, which works by changing brain chemistry to convince the body it is not hungry. Xenical or Alli is approved for children 12 and older, which is formulated to stop the absorption of fat that comes from consumed food.

Surgery

In addition to diet, exercise, and modified behavior, doctors may suggest other treatments for child obesity. Although there are reported cases of teenagers having surgery in the fight against obesity, reputable doctors would never perform a serious surgery such as Gastric Bypass on a small child. In fact, even when used for older children, the decision to perform surgery is complex.

We are now seeing a greater number of highly qualified surgeons offering the Lap Band or Gastric Bypass surgery to older teenagers. Of course, any type of invasive procedure such as surgery would only be a consideration in extreme cases of obesity and even then, the child would be required to meet very strict requirements and both child and parents would have to understand potential risks involved.

For the teenager with obesity that had tried all the traditional treatment options and given 100% effort to losing weight but without any or much success, surgery might be a consideration. However, because there are no long-term studies to show how the Lap Band or Gastric Bypass surgery affects a child's growth and development, the decision to go forward is difficult.

The most important thing is for the parents to talk to a number of board-certified surgeons first so all pros and cons could be understood and weighed against the expected outcome. If at any time a parent were to meet with a surgeon eager to do the surgery without taking the required time to examine the child and understand his or her history, they should run out of the office as quickly as possible.

ADOPTING A HEALTHY LIFESTYLE

Along with getting the proper medical intervention and treatment, a lot of the responsibility for dealing with child obesity falls back on the parents. After all, the child needs to adopt a healthy lifestyle in coordination with support offered by the doctor.

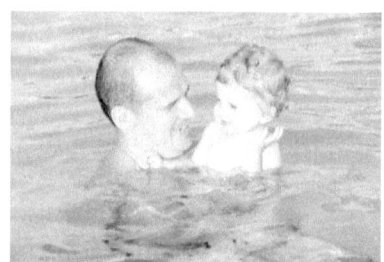

We have mentioned throughout the book the importance of the entire family getting onboard in treating an obese child but we cannot stress enough how the journey of preventing and managing child obesity as a team is far more successful.

Healthy Eating

Starting with food again, as a parent you are the one that actually goes to the grocery store, buys the food, and brings it home to prepare for everyone to eat. Therefore, change regarding eating habits must begin with you. Something that many parents do not realize is that making even small changes can have big results. The following are some recommendations for making change.

- Choose fresh fruits and vegetables instead of canned. The reason is that most canned fruits are loaded with unnecessary sugar and canned vegetables are packed with sodium (salt) that an obese child does not need.

- Avoid buying soda and high-sugar fruit juices, choosing low calorie beverages instead. For instance, instead of buying prepared lemonade in the store, you could make a healthier version at home using fresh lemons, ice, water, and a sugar substitute.
- Provide snack time for your child but never use food as a reward or for a punishment
- Always enjoy meals as a family unit. Studies show families that sit at the table to eat together experience fewer incidences of child suicide, which shows the power that family dinner time has. Never allow anyone in the family to eat in front of the television or while playing/working on the computer.
- Enjoy dining out on occasion but not more than once or twice a month. Even then, try to choose restaurants that offer health menu selections. This way, the child does not feel deprived and after eating low calorie, well-balanced meals at home, he or she has something special to look forward to when going out.

A key contributor to child obesity is fast and processed foods . . .

. . . Avoid them at all cost!

Get Moving

Regarding physical activity, remember to establish time for family fun. This could be something as simple as going for a walk after dinner, heading to the nearest YMCA or gym to swim or workout, taking a bike ride on a Saturday afternoon, and so on. In addition to helping the obese child lose weight, daily exercise in one form or another helps build strong bones and muscles that children need.

Once the entire family gets moving with some kind of physical activity, everyone will sleep better, find it easier to concentrate, and experience fewer bouts of depression or irritability. The truth is that physical activity is an excellent tool for physical health but also mental and emotional health. Tips for getting an obese child interested in something physical include:

- Computer, Television, and Games—You do not have to eliminate computer, television, and game time altogether but it would be highly beneficial to establish a schedule or exact number of hours the child could spend on these activities. At first, the child may feel frustrated and angry, or even as if being punished but introducing healthier activities will help the child adjust.

- Stop Exercising—No child wants to be told that he or she has to start "exercising". Instead, introduce the concept of "physical activity", which involves family fun, but specifically an activity that would interest the child.
- Fun Activities—The best way to get an obese child involved in physical activity is to allow him or her to choose. You could certainly offer some age-appropriate suggestions but then allow your child to decide. By doing this, the child will be more eager to get started, as well as appreciate being provided with some independence.
- Family Participation—We cannot stress this enough—if the obese child is going to be encouraged to participate in a physical activity, everyone in the family should get onboard. This provides needed support to the child but also provides the entire family with an opportunity to get and stay healthy while bonding.
- Mix Things Up—Children, especially small children become bored and disinterested quickly so to keep their attention, it is important to mix things up regarding physical activity. For instance, you could sign the family up for three months of martial arts and if the child began to show disinterest, try gymnastics, swimming, etc.

HEALTHY DIET PLANS

When creating a healthy diet plan for your obese child there are ways of making this succeed or fail. In this chapter, we wanted to provide information and helpful tips specific to diet plans for the child living with obesity.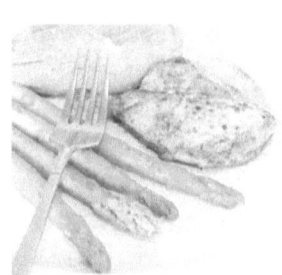

Food is such a huge part of the problem that you literally have to start over, teaching the child the right way to eat. This process takes time and effort but with determination and perseverance, your child will soon enjoy the new and healthy diet plan.

Tips for a Successful Diet

The following are excellent tips to get the new diet plan off the ground and to keep your obese child interested.

- Provide well-balanced meals but without excessive restrictions. Especially when first making changes, you do not want to cut everything out. For instance, if your child is accustomed to dessert with dinner each night, go ahead and offer him or her a piece of cake or pie, but reduce the size by 50% and consider making dessert with a sugar substitute so it has fewer calories.
- Make sure meals are properly balanced to include all major food groups—fresh fruits and vegetables, lean meats, whole grains, and low-fat dairy products. After all, whether obese or not, children

require vitamins and minerals for proper growth and development that are found in all food groups.

- To spice up otherwise bland food, switch to healthy ingredients. For instance, oatmeal is a great breakfast food but instead of adding butter and brown sugar, it could be flavored with honey or fresh fruit.
- Think outside the box when it comes to lunch. Throwing together a peanut butter and jelly sandwich or driving through a fast food restaurant is easier and faster but it also adds to the problem of obesity. A better choice would be healthy foods your child likes such as a baked potato spruced up with low-fat cheese, fresh steamed broccoli, and a mild salsa or homemade macaroni and cheese made with low-fat cheese and milk and wholegrain coupled with mixed steamed vegetables.
- Even for dinner, simple changes would make a big difference. As an example, instead of fixing standard spaghetti and garlic bread, make the meal with whole grain spaghetti, homemade sauce made with fresh vegetables, and add a cup of diced fresh fruit on the side.
- Everyone loves dessert, especially children but you have to eliminate cakes, pies, cookies, and other traditional choices. Now, an occasional small piece would be fine but ultimately, the goal would be to serve healthier desserts such as low-fat frozen yogurt topped with a dollop of low-fat whipped cream and fresh fruit or low calorie pudding mixed with pieces of fresh fruit.
- Offer healthy choice snacks such as raisins, yogurt covered pretzels, crackers with natural peanut butter, fresh fruit smoothie, or cup of yogurt.
- Both salt and fat levels need to be reduced. Although needed by the body to function properly most children consume far too much and for obese children, salt and fat are the enemies.
- If you cannot come up with a workable diet plan, you can always sit down with the doctor that treats your child or meet with a licensed dietician or nutritionist. Remember, even when a child is obese, without a proper diet, malnutrition is possible. Therefore, the child needs to get the appropriate number of calories but from healthier food choices.
- If you decide to go with an established diet plan such as South Beach, Atkins, or The Zone, etc, always run it by the doctor first. Some of these diets are good considerations for an obese child but

because there are so many dynamics, only the treating doctor could determine if any should be used.

- Allow the child to participate in shopping and cooking processes. Remember, treating obesity is about education, not just for parents but also the children. Therefore, teaching a child about healthy foods by allowing participation in the shopping and cooking process would be beneficial.

MANAGEMENT TIPS

After an obese child has dropped the weight and gone through behavioral modification, now what. Obviously, getting the weight off was the biggest obstacle but because the child experienced obesity, the potential for putting the weight back on by going back to old habits is always possible.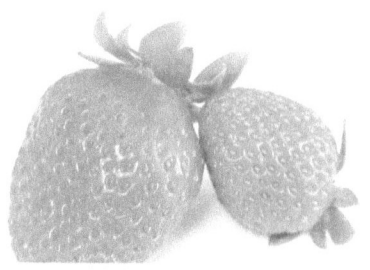

While it might sound harsh, even after the child has dropped the weight, child obesity is a lifelong issue. Unless children stay focused and have the appropriate tools and resources to continue on the path of success, some will eventually revert to their old ways and before long, find themselves living as an obese adult. As you have probably heard a thousand times, proper eating is not about being on a "diet" but about making healthy food choices.

As a parent, you have the remarkable opportunity to moderate food consumption to help your child stay at the appropriate weight. With this, your child's level of self-esteem and confidence will increase and before long, his or her outlook on life will be very different. Remember, psychological challenges are commonly linked to child obesity so as a part of the management program you can boost your child's attitude so he or she can accomplish whatever goal lies ahead.

Strategies for Maintaining Weight

In this section, we have provided some management tools that parents and children can use to maintain a healthy weight once the battle of losing weight is over.

- Start a weight management program
- Stick to a routine of eating healthy, consuming smaller portions, and eating slowly so food can digest properly
- Develop a meal plan to make shopping and preparation easier
- Establish a physical activity schedule for six months out
- Get involved with a support group

Maintaining Goals

The following steps have long been used for management of post-obesity. In addition to educating the child and the rest of the family what it will take to help the child continue living healthy and happy, you might even consider creating a poster and hang it where everyone can see it daily as a gentle reminder of goals and accomplishments.

1. Medical—Parents working with the child's doctor to make sure regular check-ups are followed up on is a huge benefit.
2. Education—A part of any good management plan is the aspect of ongoing education
3. Environment—Making appropriate changes in the home such as removing all junk food, putting limitations on television, computer, and video game playing, and finally, scheduling family time for fitness are imperative to continued success
4. Behavior—Even after the child has completed behavior modification, intermittent check-ups is advised
5. Support—Today, excellent support groups exist for children living with and getting past obesity, which is highly recommended
6. Invest in a Body Mass Index calculator, which is a diagnostic tool that can be used at home to monitor the child's BMI

Avoiding the Obesity Trap

For preventing obesity and managing a child's post-obesity weight, it is crucial not to become trapped. As you will see from the list below, avoiding the child obesity trap is actually easy. These responsibilities are for parents, as well as grandparents, siblings, and other family members, as well as teachers, counselors, and other leaders in the community.

- Role Model—Be a role model since children naturally follow what they are taught
- Provide Support—Obese children are smart and know they are different from most other children. Therefore, these children do not need to be reminded they have a weight problem but instead, supported with acceptance, unconditional love, encouragement, education, and even friendship.
- Establish Guidelines—As mentioned throughout this book, it is imperative that you set guidelines. The child is going to have a hard time at first but soon, he or she will understand the limited television, healthier snacks, and other changes are to benefit, not to harm.
- Plan Activities—Again, we cannot stress enough the value that comes out of the entire family participating in physical activity, no matter how big or small.
- Show Sensitivity—Obese children deal with stares, rude remarks, and teasing all day long so the last thing they need is to come home to a safe haven only to be embarrassed. Sometimes, innocent comments are made that to a child without obesity would think nothing of but because the obese child is far more sensitive, you as the parent and other family members need to show sensitivity to the child.
- Eat Together—This is another important tip for handling obesity. Family dinner is more than just sitting down at the table to eat. This time provides the opportunity to bond, a time for children to share things about the day's events, voice concerns, tell a funny story, and simply let their guard down without worrying about repercussions.
- Stay Prepared—You know your child is going to come home after school and snack and if the child had an exceptionally difficult time, the need to use food for comfort is going to be overwhelming.

To help, keep healthy snacks stocked. This could include frozen yogurt or pure juice bars, cut up fruits and vegetables kept in a glass of water in the refrigerator, vanilla wafers or gingersnaps, yogurt, frozen grapes, etc.

- Remain Focused—It is also important to stay focused on goals, as well as recognize what things are working and what things need to be modified.
- Celebrate—Take time to recognize small accomplishments, followed by acknowledging them. With child obesity, looking too far into the future would overwhelm everyone. Instead, set small goals and when achieved, celebrate.

HELPFUL RESOURCES

In this chapter, parents will find numerous resources to make living with and supporting an obese child easier and more effective. Parents need to remember that most children dealing with this condition also struggle with psychological issues so sometimes the journey to recovery can be long and challenged.

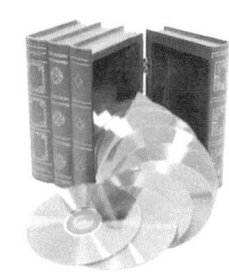

Using any of these resources can reduce stress involved and provide incredible information that can be used by the parents and the child.

Books

The following books are exceptional reads, some that can benefit the parents and child and some just for the child, or for mom and dad.

Proper Nutrition

Because poor diet is one of the primary causes of child obesity, we wanted to put it first on our list of suggested resources. Any of the following books would provide information about good nutrition that the entire family can benefit from, whether overweight or obese. These books would be ideal to prevent a child from becoming obese or helping one already obese.

- Trim Kids—This book offers a 12-week plan that uses a combination of nutrition, exercise, and behavior modification to help children lose and control weight

- Underage and Overweight—This 7-step diet and exercise plan is exceptional, teaching both parents and children how to adopt a healthy lifestyle
- Slim and Fit Kids—With fast food being such a huge problem, this book helps parents develop a sound dietary plan for their overweight or obese child
- AAP Guide to your Child's Nutrition—With this, parents can build healthy eating habits for their child and other family members, lessons that can be used throughout life

Physical Activity

As mentioned, choosing a physical activity that interests the child and one that the entire family can do together is always the best course of action. Along with the few ideas we provided earlier in this book, the following publications will expand your options.

- 365 Activities for Fitness, Food, and Fun for the Whole Family—Loaded with great eating and exercise ideas, this is a book that every parent of an obese child should own.
- 2008 Physical Activity Guidelines for Americans—This publication is offered by the US government and found at http://www.health. gov/paguidelines/guidelines/default.aspx#toc.
- Physical Activity Interventions in Children and Adolescents—This book was written to promote physical activity for children of varying ages.
- Beyond the Gym—To help fight the problem of child obesity, this book offers ideas for physical activities but also lesson plans that cover 36 weeks.
- Physical Activity and Obesity Book—This comprehensive book addresses ways to modify physical activities of children with obesity.

Behavior Modification

As we discussed, obese children often struggle with self-image issues. The older the child becomes while being heavy the more intense the problem can be. The way in which children deal with self-confidence and self-esteem issues varies.

Some children become very withdrawn and shy, actually learning to fear being in social settings, some become very angry, blaming the world for all the teasing endured, and some become over achievers, trying desperately to prove their self-worth.

Regardless of how a child responds to living a life of obesity, behavior modification is needed. This helps realign the child's thinking to how a non-obese child would think. Many excellent books exist that can help parents learn the appropriate way to deal with an obese child, as well as teach the child how to not be a victim but a victor.

- Prevention and Treatment of Childhood Obesity—The great thing about this book is that if provides a number of clinical models specific to evaluation and treatment of obesity. The book also outlines the role doctors should take, appropriate diet and activity, and behavior modification techniques.
- Progress in Behavior Modification: Volume 10—In this book, parents and obese children can read about the assessment of social skills, statistics for evaluating, measuring, and treating obesity, behavior treatment, progressive relaxation techniques, and psychopharmacological support for behavior modification.
- Understanding Childhood Obesity—With this, parents can learn about a number of prevention strategies, new and innovative treatment options, and behavior modification techniques specific to child obesity.

Just for Kids

These books are written specifically for children with obesity on their level as an educational tool.

- Too Much (Focus Focus Focus)—For children four to eight, this book features bright and fun illustrations and text that is rhyming and engaging. The storyline is about an obese boy named Luke, which allows the reader to follow his story as he learns to eat right and exercise more.
- Oscar & Otis: Fat Fighters—Also for children between ages four and eight, this book is about two friends that learn about proper

nutrition and exercise together, as they try to help one of the father's battle excessive weight.

- Just for Kids—For the pre-teen and teenager living with obesity, this workbook is great. The obesity prevention program is easy to follow and designed to teach children about healthy lifestyle choices.
- Fat Tale—This book is also for the pre-teen and teenager that deals with obesity. This picture book focuses primarily on good nutrition, helping to educate kids about the consequences of poor eating.

Parental Support

Being the parent of an obese child is often more difficult than being the child. Obviously, parents have a built-in protection measure when it comes to children. Watching a child struggle with making friends, dealing with school, or trying to fit into various social settings but being rejected because of obesity is heartbreaking.

As you and your child work toward a healthier life, you too need support because you will have to be strong for your child and a great example. The following books are recommended solely for parents to help them cope during this journey.

- Our Overweight Children: What Parents, Schools, and Communities Can do to Control the Fatness Epidemic—The great thing about this particular book is that it was written not just for parents of obese children but also school officials and communities. The unique approach of dealing with child obesity as a unit has been proven extremely effective.
- Rescuing the Emotional Lives of Overweight Children—The advice provided in this book is simple but effective. Parents will learn the right way to address and coach children to reach success in the battle against obesity.
- Child Obesity: A Parent's Guide to a Fit, Trim, and Happy Child—The last book for parents of an obese child we want to mention is this one. The great thing about this book is that it covers information whether the child is an infant or teenager.

DVDs

You will also find a number of excellent DVDs on the market developed for obese children and their parents. The following are just a few of the many DVDs we would recommend.

- Bounce 'n' Jam—Interactive, fun, bright, colorful, fun, and engaging, this DVD is outstanding and something everyone will love.
- Food Fight: Childhood Obesity and the Food Industry—Parents will learn a lot about child obesity about this ABC News DVD, which shows how the food industry uses marketing strategies that impact the children and obesity
- Life Success for Kids: Strategies for Conquering the Childhood Obesity Epidemic—This DVD is one of which the entire family can benefit. Included are tips on engaging children in the fight against obesity, eight steps for staying healthy, happy, and successful, and various facts about the causes of child obesity.

Support Groups

Regardless of where in the world you live, chances are a support group for child obesity is not far. If you cannot locate one offered through a private party, you can always contact a local hospital or talk to the child's doctor for recommendations. Of course, if a support group cannot be located for in-person meetings, online support groups are also an excellent solution.

The best way to locate a support group for child obesity is to use any of the main search engines such as Google.com, Yahoo.com, and Lycos.com, typing in keywords "support groups for child obesity" or "child obesity support groups" followed by the name of the city where you live.

You will find some excellent online groups, people just as you that need a place to vent, need advice and tips, or need someone who can understand the challenges of child obesity to celebrate with them.

www.ingramcontent.com/pod-product-compliance
Lightning Source LLC
Chambersburg PA
CBHW021259280526
45784CB00005B/2428